Most of us have a pretty good understanding of what it takes to be healthy and fit.

Three things. We know that we should eat right, get regular exercise, and avoid harmful substances.

In broad, general terms, **we get it.**

Here's the real problem:
People aren't good at reshaping their habits.

Nobody's against wellness. Everyone *wants* to be in top physical condition. **Trouble is, that's not enough.**

So what's the answer?

Solution #1: Learn how to change.

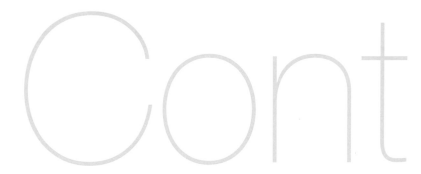

International rights and foreign translations available only through negotiation with PRITCHETT.

Printed in the United States of America

ISBN 978-0-944002-75-9

ents

Five Realities of Wellness and Work

1. Your Health Habits Are Part of Your Work Habits.
2. Wellness Is a Measure of Your Worth to the Organization.
3. Fitness Maximizes Your Energy and Quality of Life.
4. The Absence of Illness Isn't Proof of Wellness.
5. Your Body Reports to You.

Live in the Strike Zone for Fitness and Health

6. Shape Your Eating Habits for the 21st Century.
7. Work Up a Sweat Every Day.
8. Program Two Kinds of Exercise into Your Life.
9. Monitor Your Weight.
10. Stay Away from Harmful Substances.

Solution #1: Learn How to Change

11. Aim Your Brain Toward Wellness.
12. Build Psychological Muscle.
13. Practice the "60-Second Commitment."
14. Don't Misinterpret Your Moments of Truth.
15. Ritualize the Big Payoff Behaviors.

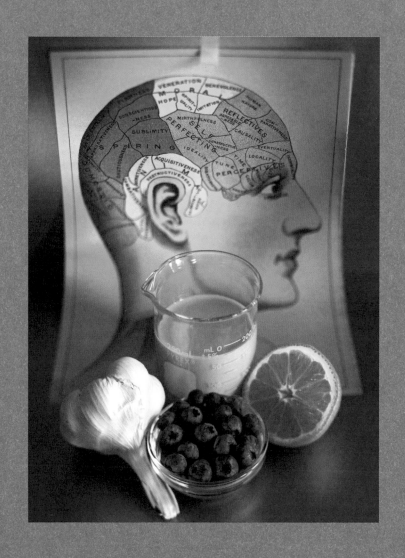

Five Realities of
Wellness and Work

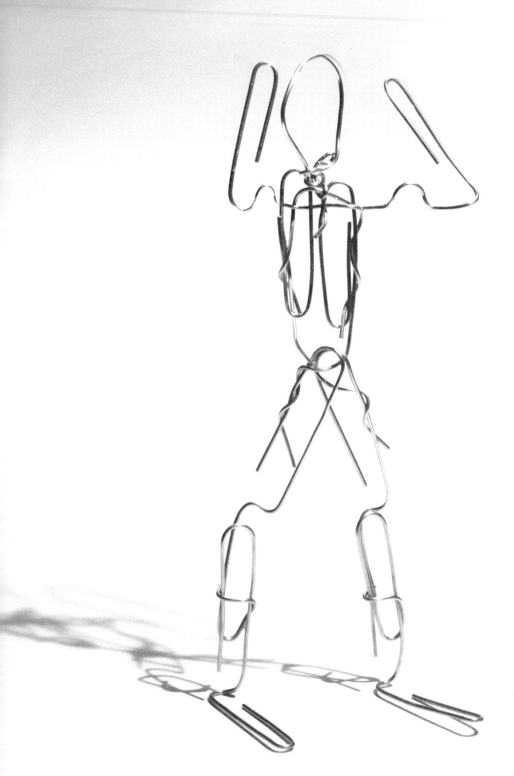

3

Your Health Habits Are Part of Your Work Habits.

You may not have thought of it this way, but managing your personal health and fitness is a job skill.

Why? Because you always bring your health to work. It affects the way you do your job—for better or for worse—and can matter every bit as much as your abilities, education, and experience.

Your body and mind are part of the equipment you work with. If this equipment is in poor shape, it hurts your performance. If you're in excellent health, it helps you perform up to your full potential.

Whether we like it or not, our health habits are part of our work habits, because they directly influence our job effectiveness.

So take care of yourself because it positions you to do your best work.

Forbes.com reported recently that health benefits now represent more than 7% of payroll costs for firms. And research shows that most of the costs of rising health premiums will ultimately come out of the employees' wages.

Here's the key point: You *personally* have a financial stake in your coworkers' wellness.

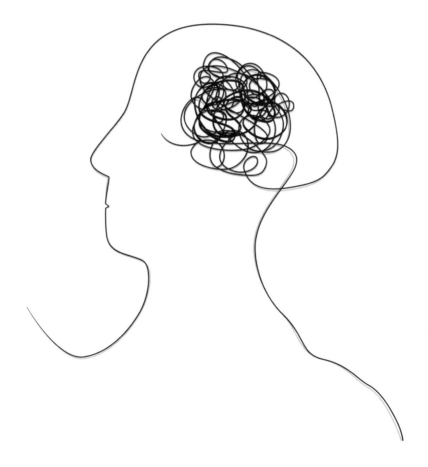

"It takes six months to get into shape and two weeks to get out of shape. Once you know this you can stop being angry about other things in life and only be angry about this."

—Rita Rudner

2

Wellness Is a Measure of Your Worth
to the Organization.

Your health is not simply a personal matter. It's also a serious business issue, because it directly affects profitability.

Health problems make insurance more expensive for everyone. They also weaken overall productivity, and that's another drain on the company pocketbook.

Your wellness matters because the company has money on the line. Healthcare issues are a big part of the cost structure, and it's your responsibility to help keep these expenses under control.

In fact, keeping your health in top shape can be as important as staying sharp in your technical skills.

It might make you angry, or hit you as unfair, but here's the reality: Everything else being equal, people who make the effort to keep themselves healthy and fit are worth more than employees who don't manage themselves toward wellness.

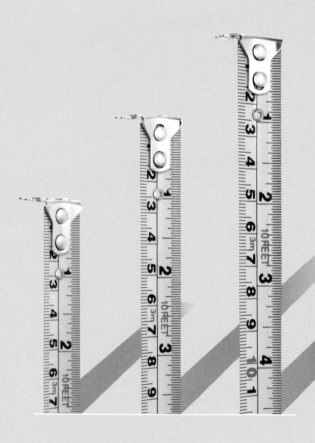

" You can't lose weight without exercise. But I've got a philosophy about exercise. I don't think you should punish your legs for something your mouth did. Drag your lips around the block once or twice.   —Gary Owens "

The costs of people being overweight and obese increase the annual medical bill by more than

$90,000,000,000

per year. You and other taxpayers foot the bill for about half of this through Medicare and Medicaid coverage.

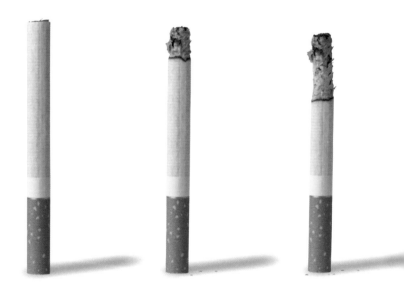

Health Affairs reports that obese individuals spend about 36% more than the general population on health services and 77% more on medications.

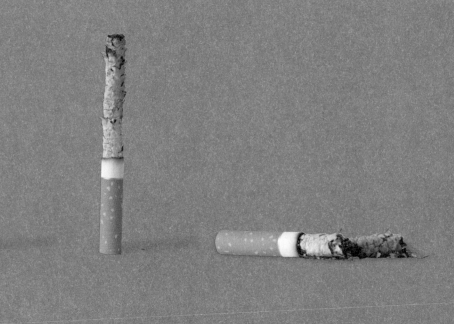

IN FACT, the effects of obesity on health spending significantly outpace the effects of current or past smoking.

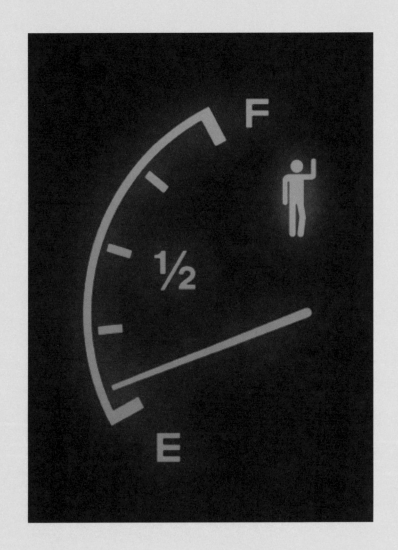

3

Fitness Maximizes Your Energy and Quality of Life.

"Getting in shape" is one of the greatest gifts you can give to yourself.

Fitness is the magnificent enabler, the life-expanding state that blows open your world of possibilities and adds richness to all your experiences. Like a broad-spectrum antibiotic, being in shape makes everything better. The benefits go far beyond the physical realm, oozing deep into the psychological, social, and professional aspects of your being.

Energy, defined as "the capacity to do work," is the natural by-product of fitness. If you're poorly conditioned, there's a shortage of this juice for you to use on the job. You also run low on fuel in your personal time. Body and spirit both suffer for lack of fire power.

For most of us, fitness requires deliberate effort. Some sacrifice. But it's an act of kindness toward ourselves, and it becomes self-reinforcing. Give yourself a chance to get hooked on healthy.

 All God's children are not beautiful. Most of God's children are, in fact, barely presentable.   —Fran Lebowitz

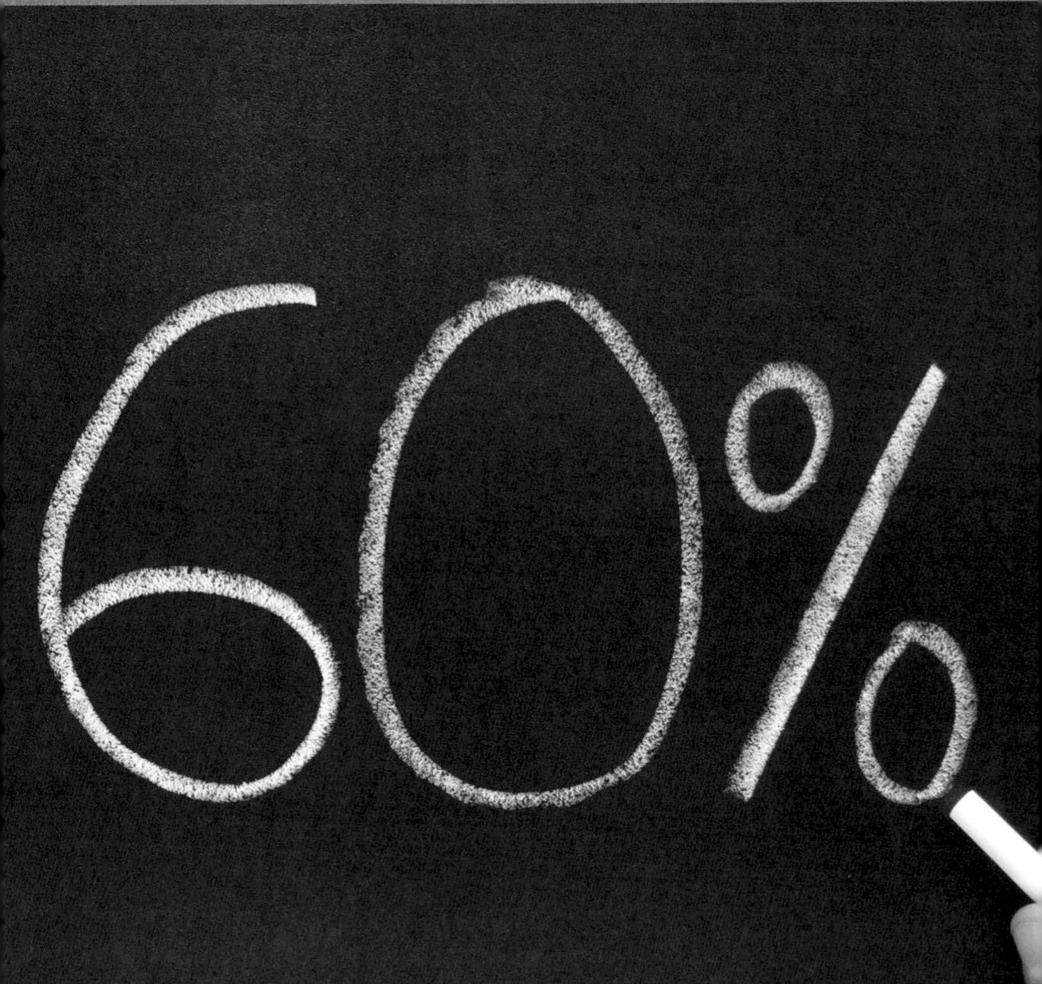
60%

"More than 60% of Americans are
overweight or obese;
127 million people are overweight,
60 million are obese, and
9 million are severely obese."

"American adults are now, on average, **25 pounds heavier**
than they were in **19**60."

—David Shields,
*The Thing About Life Is That One Day
You'll Be Dead*

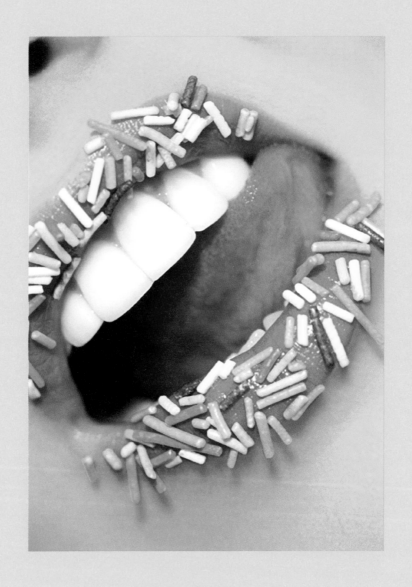

4

The Absence of Illness Isn't Proof of Wellness.

You don't have to be sick to have serious health problems. And even if you feel okay you can be in poor physical condition.

Millions of people are living with dangerous risk factors that make them an easy target for life-threatening disease. Even more people are so out of shape that it hurts their quality of life, weakens their performance, and leaves them vulnerable to the next bug that comes along.

You need to shoot for more than just not being sick.

Aim toward wellness, because it represents a higher standard of health. Wellness is about playing in the zone of prevention—consciously avoiding the common hazards and following the practices of positive health.

Pay attention to the trend lines in your personal health and fitness. And keep improving.

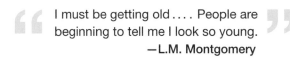

" I must be getting old .... People are beginning to tell me I look so young.
—L.M. Montgomery

In *Beating Cancer with Nutrition*, author Patrick Quillin states,

"Only 42% of Americans will actually develop detectable cancer, yet most experts agree that everyone gets cancer about six times per lifetime with one cancer cell sprouting up in everyone each day."

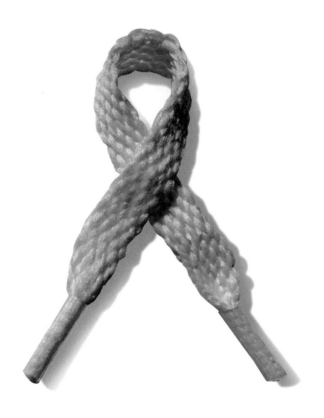

"It is the surveillance of an alert and capable immune system that defends most of us from cancer .... Only 14% of active Americans will get cancer .... A half-hour of exercise every other day cuts the risk of breast cancer by 75%."

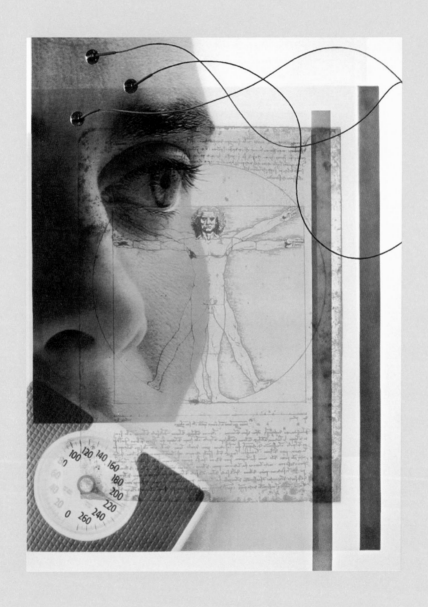

5

Your Body Reports to You.

Everyone in the organization has management responsibilities: You're the boss of your body … the supervisor in charge of your behavior … the decision-maker who's personally accountable for your fitness and health.

Wellness is a self-management issue.

Granted, you might inherit bad genes. You could be a victim of circumstances and get hit by some random illness or accident. Maybe your personal situation makes it tough for you to take good care of yourself. But how you deal with such unwelcome situations remains a personal choice.

Regardless of what life deals us, our responsibility is to do what we personally can to protect our health. We can't escape the fact that we're each in charge of our overall well-being.

 How can you tell whether or not you have had enough until you've had a little too much? —Jessamyn West

Leisure time in America has increased by more than four hours per week since 1965. But about one-fourth of all adults get no physical activity at all in their leisure time.

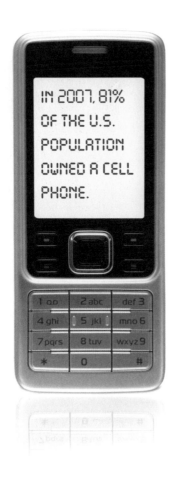

IN 2007, 81% OF THE U.S. POPULATION OWNED A CELL PHONE.

Only 15% possessed a
health club membership.

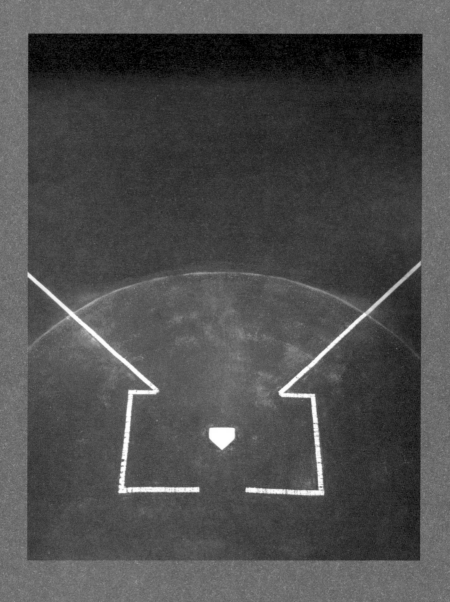

Live in the Strike Zone for Fitness and Health

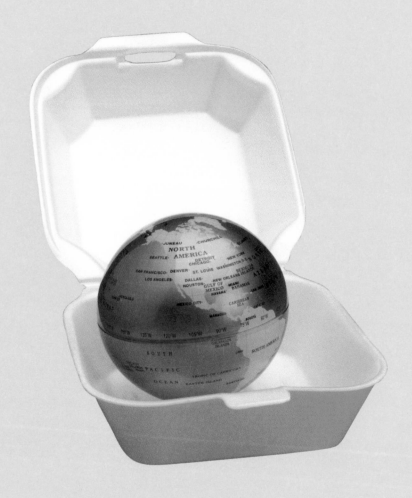

Shape Your Eating Habits for the 21ˢᵗ Century.

Never before in human history have we had so many food choices, so readily available, so cheaply. But the curses of abundance are today's major threat to wellness.

This is the Age of Plenty, and it's making people fat, lazy, and sick. These are the dangerous side effects of our success, proving that the knife of progress cuts both ways.

In ages past, the challenge was to find food or afford it. Now we face the opposite problem: finding the self-control to give the body what it needs rather than all that we can easily and enjoyably feed it. Today's challenges are to resist temptation, refuse to overindulge, and reset our eating habits toward wellness.

We need very different eating practices for the 21ˢᵗ century.

Our world has changed, giving us a profoundly different food supply. Now we have to change. Our lives depend on it.

 I'm at the age where food has taken the place of sex in my life. In fact, I've just had a mirror put over my kitchen table.   —Rodney Dangerfield

Worldwide, there are now more people who are overweight than undernourished.

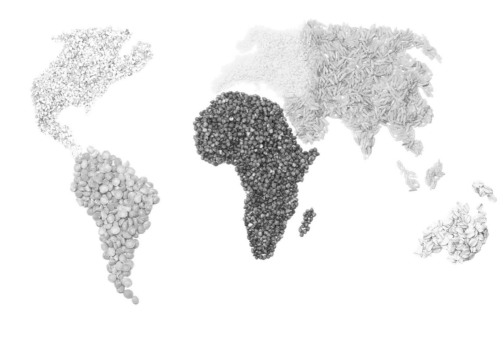

In this country, between 1971 and 2000 …

men's calorie intake grew 7%

7% ♂

and women's grew 22%.

22% ♀

idleness & ease

are the new

Killers

Work Up a Sweat Every Day.

The amazing technology gains over the past century have left us in a funny position. We've removed so much effort from everyday life that our health is seriously threatened. Idleness and ease are the new killers.

We've outsourced exertion to machines. Modern conveniences and high-tech ways free us from countless activities and physically demanding tasks. But our bones, muscles, and body chemistry—finely tuned for survival over the past half million years—weren't designed for today's sedentary lifestyle.

Human beings simply aren't engineered for the "easiness" of the modern world. We're going soft, clogging up inside, dying from under-exertion.

The only antidote is exercise. So crank up your activity level.

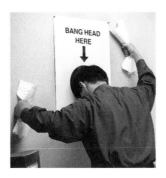

" Banging your head against a wall uses an estimated 150 calories an hour.
—Unknown "

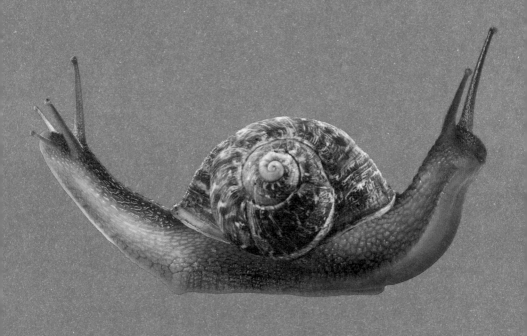

"We are not tired at the end of the day because we get too much exercise. We are tired because we do not get *enough* exercise. We are mentally, emotionally and physically drained from being sedentary."

—Chris Crowley & Henry S. Lodge, M.D.,
Younger Next Year

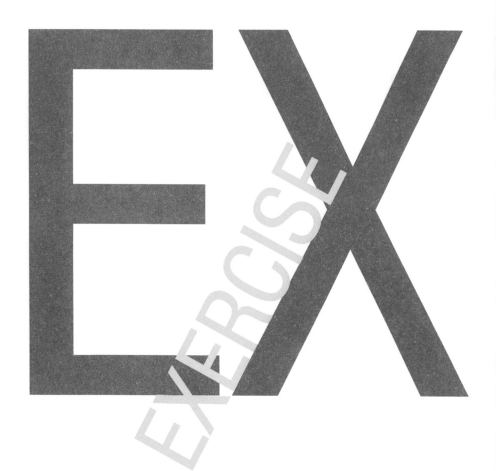

is the *single* most **powerful tool**

you have to **optimize**

your **brain function**.

—John J. Ratey, M.D., with Eric Hagerman,
Spark: The Revolutionary New Science of Exercise and the Brain

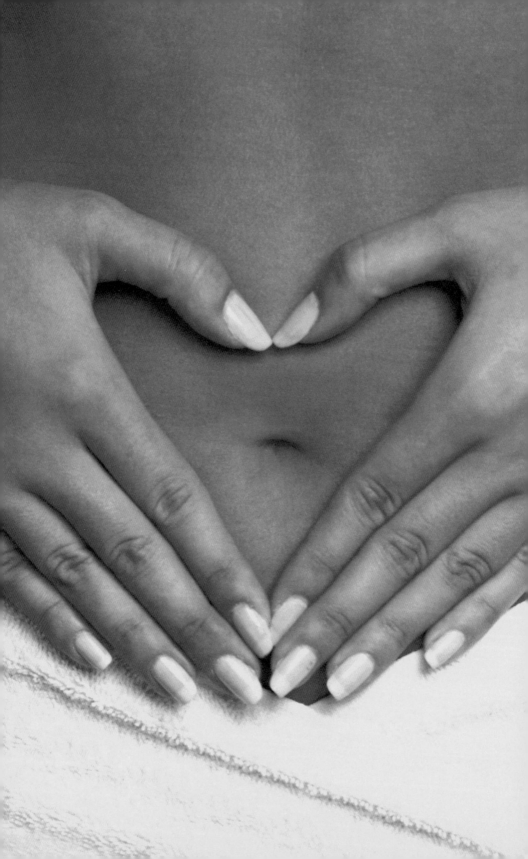

Program Two Kinds of Exercise into Your Life.

The body needs both aerobic activity and strength training. Regularly.

The first protects the heart and its plumbing; the other builds muscle and bones. Together they strengthen your immune system, pump up your energy level, reduce the chance of accidents, and enhance performance.

You won't get enough exercise from your job and daily routines. Shoot for 30 to 45 minutes of aerobics three or four times a week to ratchet up your heart rate. You can bike, jog, walk, or swim, but an ambling golf game or a lazy stroll through the mall won't cut it. Next, do strength training two or three times a week, resistance exercises like weightlifting, push-ups, and sit-ups.

Think exercise takes too much time or energy? Nope. It'll make you more productive and give you greater energy. It's also the single best thing you can do to reduce stress, lose weight, and stay young.

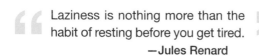

Laziness is nothing more than the habit of resting before you get tired.
—Jules Renard

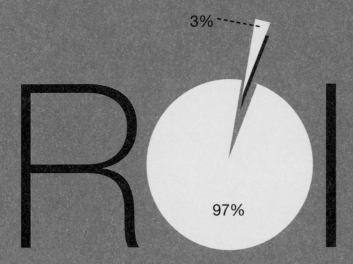

"As little as 20-30 minutes [of exercise] most days of the week is all you need to be doing to see results. That's less than 3% of your waking day, and you'll feel better for the other 97%. Think about it … that is a great return on investment."

—Christopher Bergland,
The Athlete's Way: Sweat and the Biology of Bliss

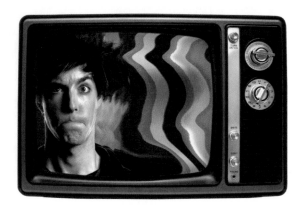

"People who watch a lot of TV are more likely to be overweight than people who don't. The less TV people watch,
the skinnier they are. It doesn't matter if they're 14 or 44."

—Brian Wansink, Ph.D.,
Mindless Eating

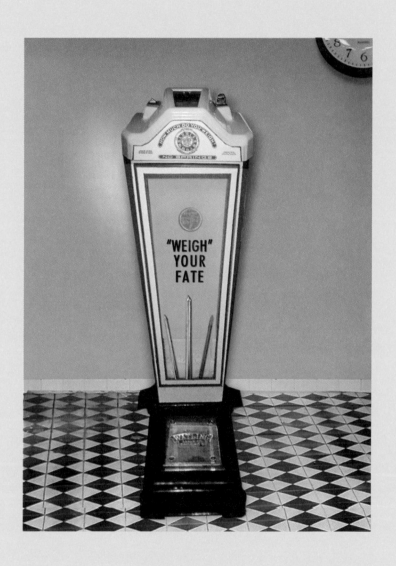

9

Monitor Your Weight.

Stepping onto the scales is like taking truth serum. It gives the lowdown on your eating and exercise habits.

Weight is a key marker of your health and fitness, a window into your current and future wellness. You need to track it … take it seriously … pay attention to what it's telling you. Every pound measured by the scales is a 3,500-calorie statement. That's about how many calories you have to burn up, or not eat, to get rid of one pound of fat.

Pretty simple.

Excess weight is a destructive, dangerous force that shouldn't be ignored.

Instead of counting on modern medicine to protect you from weight-related health problems—with a pill, stent, bypass surgery, or whatever—watch the scales. They'll tell you when to eat differently and exercise more.

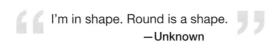
I'm in shape. Round is a shape.
—Unknown

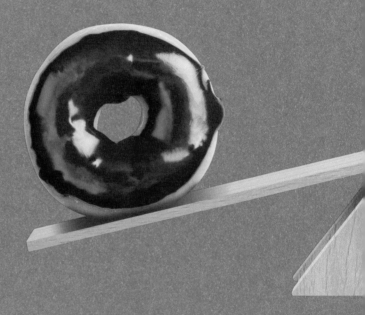

"Dieters who weigh themselves frequently tend to lose more weight."

"Ten out of the 25 most-prescribed drugs on the market today are aimed at diseases or risk factors associated with obesity."

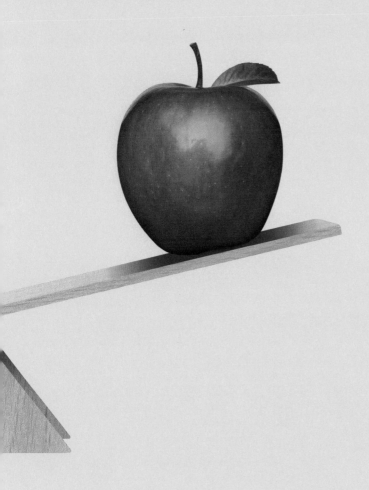

"Liposuction is the most commonly performed cosmetic surgery procedure in America. Every year over 400,000 are performed."

—Eric A. Finkelstein & Laurie Zuckerman,
The Fattening of America

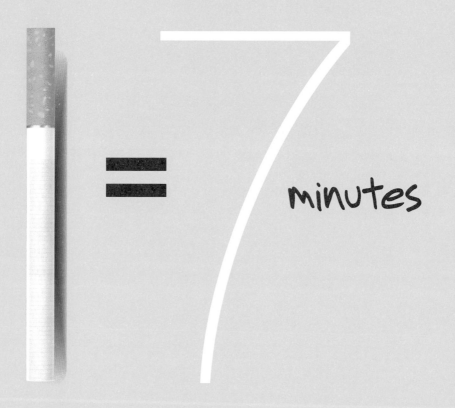

10

Stay Away from Harmful Substances.

Let's start with tobacco, which causes about 5,000,000 deaths worldwide every year. It's the only consumer product proven to kill more than half of its regular users.

Every cigarette takes seven minutes off a smoker's life. And the bystanders aren't safe either. Each year here in the United States 38,000 people die from heart disease and lung cancer caused by *passive* smoking.

So keep your distance. Some 402 billion cigarettes will be burning this year in our country.

Alcohol? Be careful there, too. Studies show that a drink or two per day may actually be beneficial. But alcohol abuse causes over 100,000 deaths in the United States and Canada each year.

 I started smoking to lose weight. After I dropped that lung, I felt pretty good.   —Michael Meehan

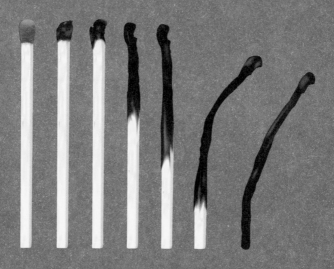

Tobacco, which killed 100 million people in the twentieth century, is on track to kill 1 billion people in the twenty-first century. Between 1997 and 2001, tobacco smoking resulted in $92 billion of annual productivity losses.

—From *The Tobacco Atlas*
　by Drs. Judith Mackay, Michael Eriksen, & Omar Shafey

"Alcohol is the third leading cause of death in the U.S."

—Drs. Kenneth H. Cooper & Tyler C. Cooper,
Start Strong, Finish Strong

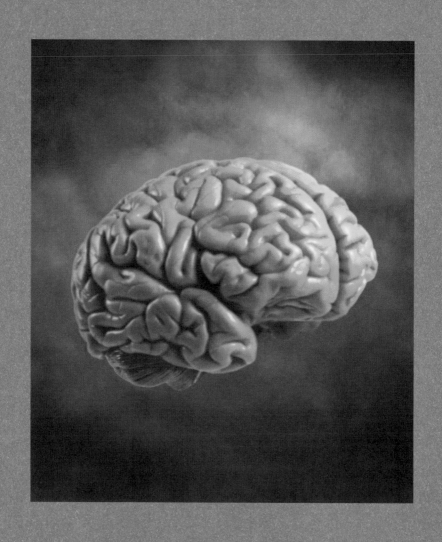

Solution #1:
Learn How to Change

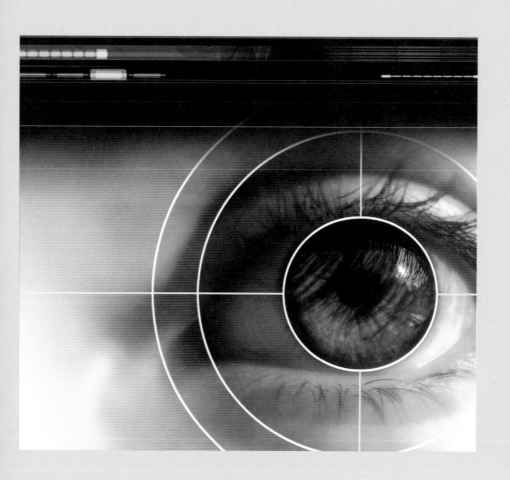

11

Aim Your Brain Toward Wellness.

The brain will be your greatest ally or your major enemy in pursuit of health and fitness. It's where most dieting and exercise efforts fail.

A key to success lies in a little bundle of cells at the base of your brain called the reticular activating system, or RAS. The RAS is a powerful homing device that can silently guide you toward health and fitness.

Here's how it works. The RAS evaluates everything you see, hear, touch, smell, or taste, searching and sorting through all incoming signals to decide what deserves your attention and what can more or less be ignored. If you make wellness a high priority in your life—if your clear intention is to become healthy and fit—the RAS navigates you in that direction. It will filter your full range of experiences, finding the ways and means to move you toward wellness.

Keep your thoughts sharply focused on the target state you seek. Wellness begins inside your head.

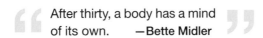

After thirty, a body has a mind of its own.   —Bette Midler

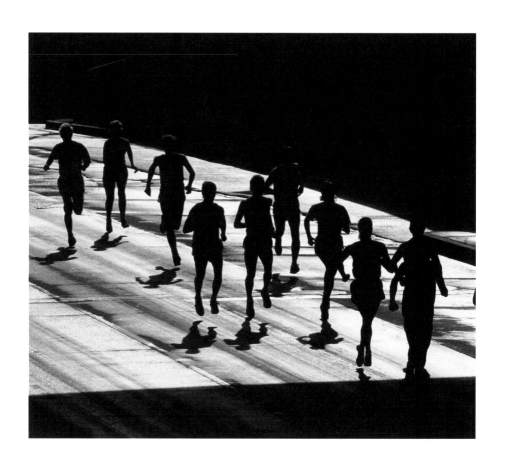

"Don't think of it as exercise. Think of it as sending a constant 'grow' message ... telling your body to get stronger, more limber, functionally younger, in the only language your body understands."

"Do it because it's the only thing that works."

—Chris Crowley & Henry S. Lodge, M.D.,
Younger Next Year

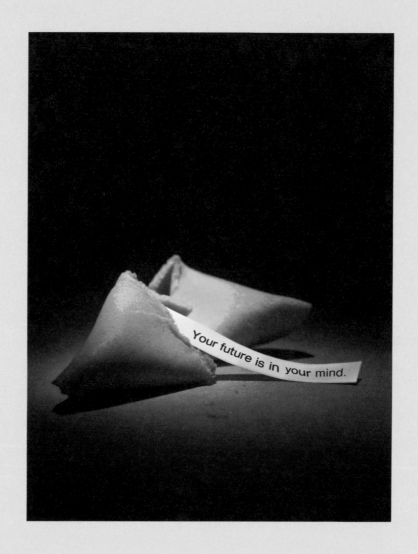

12

Build Psychological Muscle.

You need a good cheerleader to help you change your habits. And *it has to be you.*

What you think and say to yourself controls how you act and feel. The thoughts you carry in your head shape your experiences and literally help create your future.

Most people unintentionally *think* themselves into giving up on their health and fitness goals. They don't realize how crucial it is to control their self-talk. Victims of their own negativity, they gradually lose the all-important "inner game," thought by thought.

Here's what new research has found: Positive thinking is important, but *nonnegative thinking* is far more crucial. So keep your mind focused on your wellness goals—on how to get there, your progress, and the payoff. But above all, don't dwell on the negative, because that sabotages your chances for success.

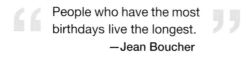

> People who have the most
> birthdays live the longest.
> —Jean Boucher

"You should think of exercise as something pleasurable that you want to do. Shift your perspective. Seek exercise, don't avoid it."

"It's a simple neural-chemical phenomenon—analgesics flood your brain in response to sweat and make you feel harmonious, centered, and euphoric."

—Christopher Bergland,
The Athlete's Way: Sweat and the Biology of Bliss

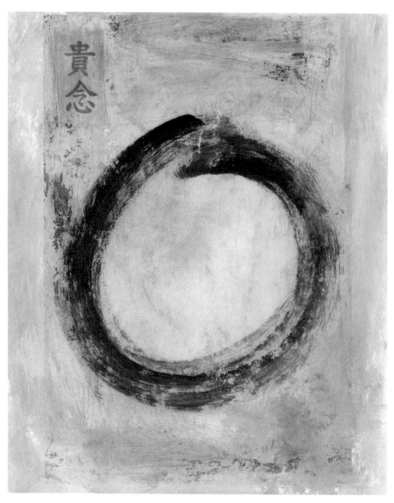

Taoist Circle of Wholeness with the Chinese characters for Noble and Thought.

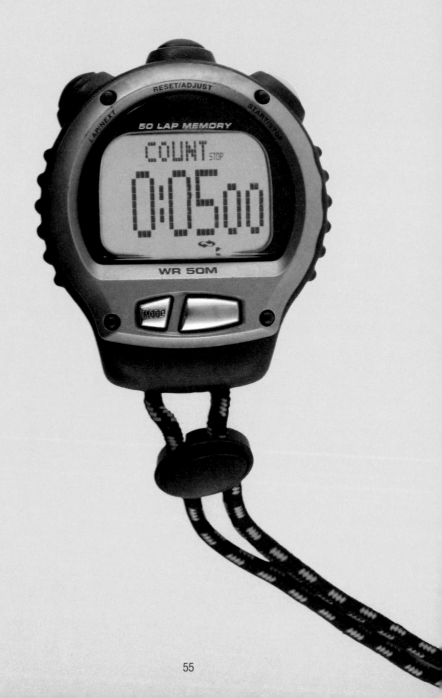

13

Practice the "60-Second Commitment."

The hardest part of a new exercise or eating routine is the first minute. It's hard to crank up for your next workout or make your next meal adhere to the new menu. But once you mobilize yourself—if you'll just discipline yourself to actually begin—the activity comes far more easily in a matter of seconds. It's sort of like the struggle one faces in trying to get up an hour earlier in the morning: *Getting up* can be difficult, but *being up* for the next 59 minutes doesn't take much effort at all.

Your challenge is to overcome inertia. Just start! Take those first steps . . . make the initial moves. Think of it as a one-minute drill that gets you over the hump and puts momentum to work for you.

Just 60 seconds of the right behavior. That's not much to ask of yourself. But if you'll make that one-minute commitment, you'll discover that you're in gear and psychologically primed to continue.

Starting is the tough part, not finishing. And the beginning is over in the blink of an eye.

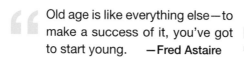

Old age is like everything else—to make a success of it, you've got to start young.   —Fred Astaire

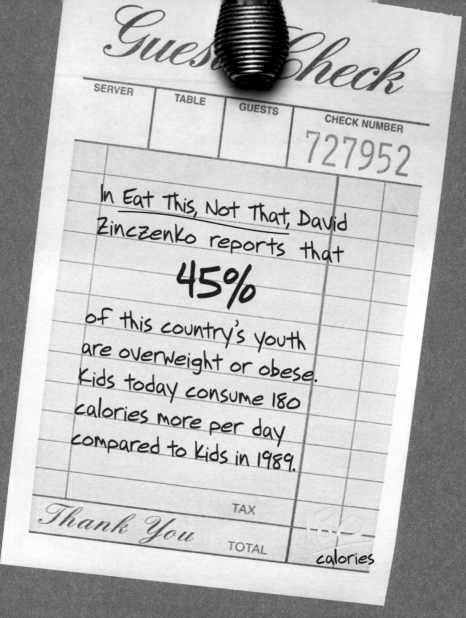

SERVER | TABLE | GUESTS | CHECK NUMBER

727952

In Eat This, Not That, David Zinczenko reports that

45%

of this country's youth are overweight or obese. Kids today consume 180 calories more per day compared to kids in 1989.

Thank You

TAX

TOTAL

180 calories

Today's epidemic of childhood obesity may reverse historical trends, causing youngsters to have a shorter life span than their parents for the first time in history.

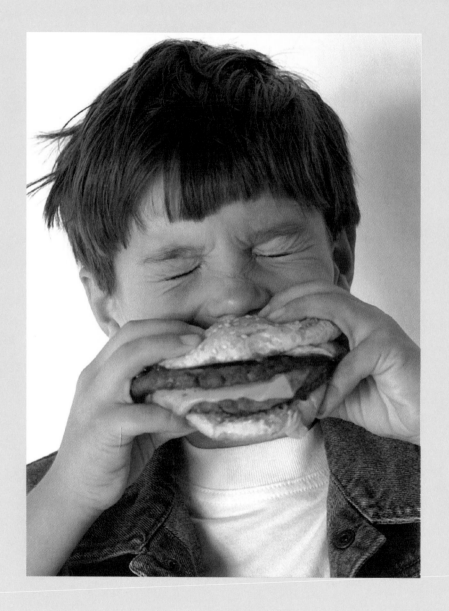

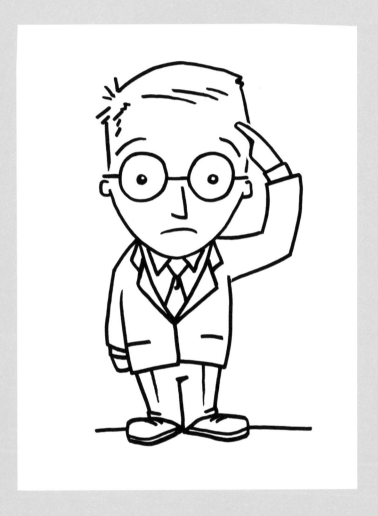

14

Don't Misinterpret Your Moments of Truth.

When you push yourself to eat better and exercise more, you hit yourself where it hurts: right smack in your habits. You violate ingrained living patterns, and something deep inside starts fighting back.

It's important for you to expect this reaction and understand the strategy of the enemy within.

Resistance to change is a great con artist. It tries to make you believe that sticking with your wellness plans will be too difficult. It wants to sweet-talk you into selling out your future for a little immediate gratification.

Don't fall for it. Sure, your new routines will make you stiff, sore, and uncomfortable at first—both psychologically and physically—but that's hard proof you're making progress. Stick with the program, and those feelings rapidly fade.

Just remember—resistance grows stronger with any evidence of weakening resolve, but it yields to renewed effort. These are the moments of truth, so hang tough.

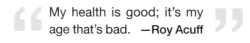

My health is good; it's my age that's bad.   —Roy Acuff

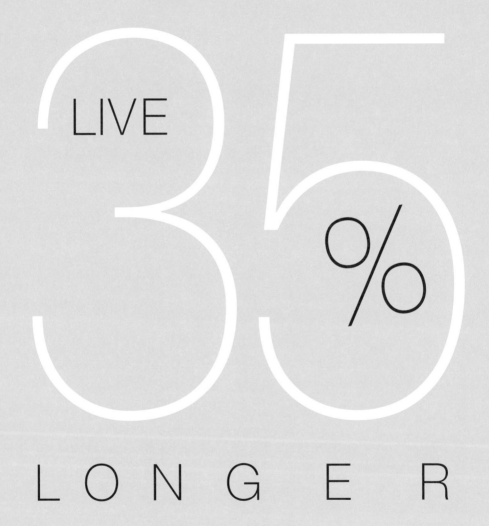

LIVE **35%** LONGER

"The truth about aging is that you—right now—have the ability to live 35% longer than expected (today's life expectancy is 75 for men and 80 for women) with a greater quality of life and without frailty."

"Restricting calories, increasing your strength, and getting quality sleep are three of nature's best anti-aging medicines."

—Drs. Michael F. Roizen & Mehmet C. Oz,
You: Staying Young

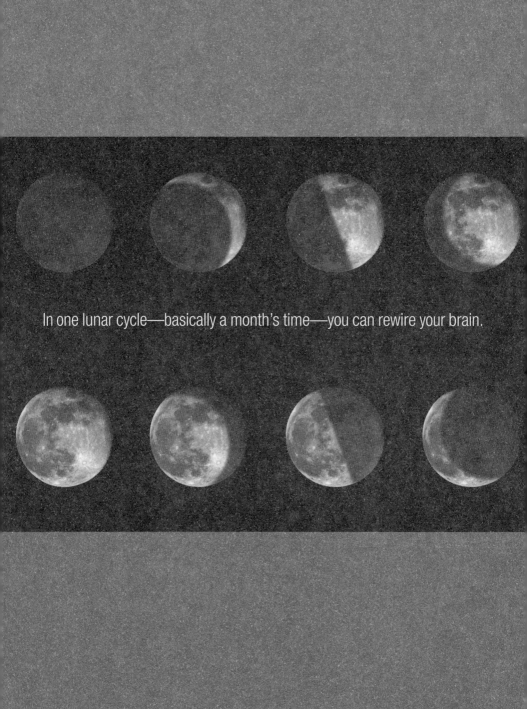

In one lunar cycle—basically a month's time—you can rewire your brain.

15

Ritualize the Big Payoff Behaviors.

Shooting for wellness may sound like a lifelong struggle. But it doesn't have to be an endless battle that relies on sacrifice and grinding self-discipline for ongoing success.

You simply need to build a few good habits. And you can develop a habit in $29^1/_2$ days.

In one lunar cycle—basically a month's time—you can rewire your brain, building new neural pathways that make wellness behavior part of your routine. The actions become ritualized, ingrained in your daily repertoire, and habit takes over. Exercising and eating right start to come naturally, like brushing your teeth or showing up for work. You do it more or less automatically.

Focus on the few changes that work the best . . . that contribute the most to wellness. Then live those big payoff behaviors religiously for $29^1/_2$ days. This is how quickly you can reach escape velocity from the gravity pull of your present living patterns.

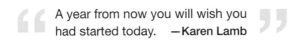

A year from now you will wish you had started today. —**Karen Lamb**

WARNING: Cigarette smoking can be detrimental to your health, but poor diet and inactivity can be worse.

"Poor diet and physical inactivity may soon overtake tobacco as the leading cause of death in America."

—Erik A. Finkelstein & Laurie Zuckerman,
The Fattening of America

"If you perform a good habit for three years, the effect on your body is as if you've done it your entire life. Even better, within three months of changing a behavior, you can start to measure a difference in your life expectancy."

—Drs. Michael F. Roizen & Mehmet C. Oz,
You: Staying Young

"No one chooses disease. It's just plain bad luck, though often piled on top of bad health.

But you choose your state of health.

You can see this as a burden or a privilege, a gift or a curse, but you can't put it down and you can't get away from it.

That's great news, if you understand the rules, because it's not that hard to take over the controls."

— Chris Crowley & Henry S. Lodge, M.D.,
Younger Next Year

Solution #1

Learn how to change.

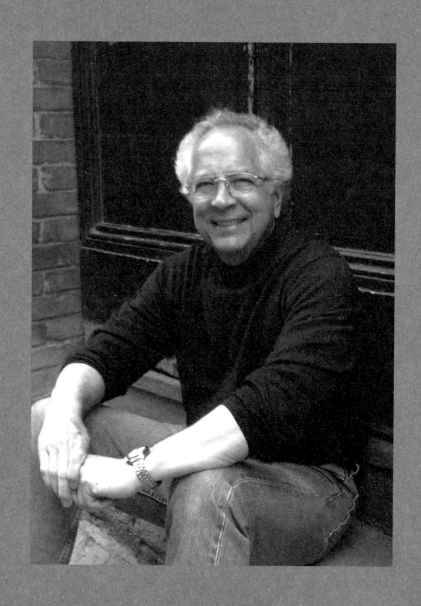

About the Author

Price Pritchett is Chairman and CEO of PRITCHETT, LP, a Dallas-based consulting and training firm with offices in seven other countries. He holds a Ph.D. in psychology and is recognized world-wide as an expert on personal and organizational change.

Dr. Pritchett's specialized work in change management, corporate culture, and merger integration has been referenced in most of the major business journals and newspapers. He also has been featured on CNN, CNBC, and other major television channels. With over 20 million copies of his books in print worldwide, he is one of the best-selling business authors in the world. Virtually all of the *Fortune* 500 companies have used some combination of PRITCHETT's consulting, training, and publications.

Books by PRITCHETT, LP

For information regarding PRITCHETT's training, keynotes, and consulting built around our handbooks, please call **800-992-5922.**

Solution #1

1-49 copies	_____ copies at $12.95 each
50-99 copies	_____ copies at $12.50 each
100-999 copies	_____ copies at $11.95 each
1,000-4,999 copies	_____ copies at $11.75 each
5,000-9,999 copies	_____ copies at $11.50 each
10,000 or more copies	_____ copies at $11.25 each

Name _____

Job Title _____

Organization _____

Address _____

City _____ State _____

Country _____ Zip Code _____

Phone _____ Fax _____

Email _____

Purchase order number (if applicable) _____

Applicable sales tax, shipping, and handling charges will be added. Prices subject to change. Orders less than $250 require prepayment. Orders of $250 or more may be invoiced. Standard shipping is FedEx 3-Day unless otherwise specified.

☐ Check Enclosed   ☐ Please Invoice

☐ **VISA**   ☐ **MasterCard**   ☐ **AMERICAN EXPRESS**

Name on Card _____

Card Number _____ Expiration Date _____

Signature _____ Date _____

PRITCHETT
DALLAS, TEXAS

For information about

Solution #1 Starter Kits

contact PRITCHETT at

800.922.5922
or www.pritchettnet.com